Reflexology

The Essential Guide for Applying Reflexology to Relieve Tension, Eliminate Anxiety, Lose Weight, and Reduce Pain

by Paula Thayer

Table of Contents

Introduction

Reflexology is an alternative type of medicine, a form of healing which involves the application of pressure or the massaging of certain points on the hands, feet and often ears, usually without the use of oil, lotion or other lubricants. This is achieved with a few specific thumb, finger and hand techniques using a recently developed modern practice that's roots are ancient, with its origins being found in many diverse cultures.

It is very difficult to determine exactly where reflexology was first used and by whom, but the first known instance of it being recorded was found in the Egyptian tomb of Ankhamor dating about 2550-BC, in the form of a pictograph. The Physicians tomb also found in Egypt dating from about the same time shows hieroglyphics that have physicians applying pressure or massaging the feet or the soles of their patients using their hands or fingers. Another example, if early reference to reflexology, can be found in a chapter in "The Yellow Emperor's Classic of Internal Medicine", a Chinese medical text book written about 1,000-BC, titled "Examining Foot Method" that is about the connections between areas on the feet and a person's life force. Other Chinese medical texts, some dating as far back as 400 BC, touted the health benefits of stimulating the hands and feet with various forms of massage, ointments, and heat. Ayurveda, a vast body of medical knowledge that originated in India, practices a type of treatment similar to reflexology. The ancient Egyptians also used a form of reflexology as far back as 2300 BC. The aboriginals of Australia a culture that has not changed for thousands of years, estimated to have first evolved 60,000 years ago also practiced their own form of reflexology. Ancient cave painting's suggest foot massage was often used to treat ailments, they claim the teachings to do this came to their medicine men through their "Dreamtime" a type of meditation and spiritual trance reached through chanting, dancing, song and other rituals. There is evidence to suggest that the native peoples of North America who had an advance form of natural medicine also engaged in foot massage to cure various ailments.

The renowned Italian world traveler Marco Polo in the 1300's translated a Chinese book that mentioned several different forms of massage including foot massage. This introduced the theory of how different parts of the body could affect others for the first time into European medicine. Doctors Adamus and A'tatis published their book called "Zone Therapy" in 1582 it is believed this is the first published European written account of what in later years would become modern reflexology Dr. Bell of Leipzig, Germany published another book on this subject about the same time.

The first time the word Reflexology was used was when it was made up by a Russian psychiatrist in the 1800's. Physicians in Russia and many Middle Eastern

Countries were widely used the application of pressure or the massaging of certain points on the hands as well as different parts of the body including the ears and head to relieve pain, discomfort, general body tension as well as for its psychological benefits. Dr. Ivan Pavlov and Dr. Vladimir Bekhterev were pioneers in the early Russian research into reflex responses in the body and their benefits. Sir Henry Head a Medical Doctor and research Scientist demonstrated that there was a link between the skin and the other body organs in the 1890's.

In the 16th century, Europe again began expanding its trade and military influence into Africa, the Middle East, and Asia. In doing so, European doctors started learning more about other forms of healing, and began incorporating a number of them into their growing repertoire of medical knowledge.

It was around this time that books were written in German and Hungarian about the topic of healing through hand and foot massage. Some of these were translated into the English language and become a fad in Britain, till they fell out of fashion due to ongoing medical advances.

Reflexology was nearly forgotten about in the English-speaking world until it was rediscovered at the turn of the last century by an ear, nose and throat specialist,

Dr. William Hope Fitzgerald, he introduced it into the United States in 1913. In 1915, a Dr. Edwin F. Bowers wrote an article for *Everybody's Magazine* entitled "To Stop That Toothache, Squeeze Your Toe".

Dr. Bowers claimed to have been studying the drug-less therapy of Dr. Fitzgerald, and praised his mentor for advancing medical science." Dr. Bowers, published a very well read articles in which he told everyone that by applying pressure to one part of the body, it was possible to ease the pain in another part. People tried Dr. Bowers' recommendations, found that they worked, and Zone Therapy became an immediate hit.

Fitzgerald called the system Zone Therapy, because he believed the body has certain "zones" that connected organs to specific areas of the body. Two years later, he co-authored the best-selling book, *Zone Therapy or Relieving Pain in the Home* with Dr. Bowers and Dr. George S. White. The publishers couldn't keep up with the demand, however, so in 1919, they came up with an enlarged and updated edition called *Zone Therapy or Curing Pain and Disease.*

It is important to note that Dr. Fitzgerald was no snake oil salesman. He earned his medical degree in 1895 from the University of Vermont, and practiced medicine at the Boston City Hospital for several years before moving to Europe.

There, he continued his medical practice, first in London, and later, in Vienna, where he worked under Dr. Ádám Politzer and Dr. Otto Chiari, the leading medical experts of their day. Returning to America, Dr. Fitzgerald became a senior surgeon at the St. Francis Hospital in Hartford, Connecticut, and was an active member of several American medical societies.

Vienna was, and still is, a leading city for medical research, having given us the likes of Carl Gustav Jung and Sigmund Freud, among others. It is therefore believed that Fitzgerald rediscovered the art of Zone Therapy during his stint in that city.

Dr. Fitzgerald had already published a number of treatises in various medical journals before portions of his work on Zone Therapy was published in *Everybody's Magazine.* Many doctors believed that his information had to be made accessible to everyone. None of them could have possibly foreseen how popular Dr. Fitzgerald's work would become, or what it would eventually lead to.

Other people took up and expanded on Dr. Fitzgerald's work, the most notable being Dr. Eunice Ingham, a trained Nurse as well as a physiotherapist. She devoted forty years of her life to the study and application of Zone Therapy, subjecting it to scientific experimentation, Dr. Ingham believed that a person's hands and feet were especially sensitive and each specific area on the hands and feet, had a direct connection with other parts of the body. Her working knowledge and experience lead her to map out what parts of the hands and feet correlate to different parts of the body, and develop the hand and foot diagrams that all Reflexologists still use today.

The first use of the word "reflexology" can be traced back to Dr. Ingham. She coined that term based on the body's involuntary "reflex" responses to certain stimuli. The methods she pioneered as well as similar techniques and methods developed by another reflexologist Laura Norman are used by many of today's Reflexologists. DR. Ingham's work was continued by her nephew, Dwight Byers, who set up the International Institute of Reflexology (http://www.reflexology-usa.net/) to preserve her work.

There is a large amount of controversy around many "Alternative Medical" techniques or health ideas. Conventional or mainstream medicine mostly refuses to accept just about all alternative forms of medicine and lobbies strongly for governments not to recognize these treatments, including reflexology. They demand that scientific evidence and physical proof be presented first, almost always refusing to accept anything outside their preferred idea of germ theory medicine and evasive practices. Despite the fact that huge numbers of people find comfort and relief using reflexology and other associated therapies that use a passive approach that considers that our body is a complete unit with all parts interconnected and working together, as well as being equipped and able to cure all ailments it would encounter in a natural world if we allowed our bodies to live naturally. Our body evolved using a wide range of naturally available foods in its hunter gather lifestyle; these foods not only nourished the body, but provided the raw materials needed for self-repair.

Many countries, including the United States consider that reflexology it is not a legitimate medical discipline. In Australia the Government's Department of Health has published the results of a review they undertook of 17 different alternative therapies, in order to determine if they had any validity for being covered by health insurance and government subsidies. Their findings were that there was no evidence of the effectiveness of reflexology and it had no effect on the human body. These findings are not surprising as these types of reviews and studies are usually partially if not fully funded by big pharma and heavily biased in their favor. Big Pharma does not like competition in any form, especially that which offers people alternatives to purchasing and using their drugs. This is very evident as other countries where big Pharma has less of a hold, have done their own studies that prove reflexology has a positive effect on people in many applications. In fact, research studies all around the world are validating the effectiveness of reflexology on a wide variety of conditions on a regular basis. Some chronic conditions that are hard to treat with conventional medicine seem to respond especially well to reflexology.

In the United Kingdom, the Complementary and Natural Healthcare Council or CNHC coordinates reflexology through a voluntary system where those registered are required to abide by the council's standards of proficiency, but this being voluntary anyone who wishes to can describe themselves as Reflexologists. Reflexologists are prevented from claiming they can provide cure for illnesses, because of a lack of factual scientific evidence that the advertising standards commission requires in order to advertise alternative treatments or therapies as a cure and the government does not recognize it as a medical service.

In Canada, the Reflexology Association of Canada has registered therapists in all provinces, but the government does not recognize them and any expenses incurred by anyone for reflexology are not eligible as a medical claim from income taxes or insurance.

In Denmark and Norway, reflexology is the most popular alternative medical treatment used. It is recognized by the national government and is integrated into the national healthcare system the United Kingdom has also recently started to recognize it officially. In China it is used together with Traditional Chinese Medicine.

Research studies, have shown that reflexology treatments and therapies have provided some improvement to 95% of the over 18,000 cases covering 64 illnesses in over 300 individual studies in China, where reflexology is accepted by the central government as a means of preventing and curing diseases and preserving health.

Several large multi-national Corporations in Japan and Denmark have been using reflexology in their health care programs with the result they have been saving thousands of dollars each year on paid out sickness benefits and saving much more because of increased productivity.

The work done by the early Reflexologists Fitzgerald and Ingham has been taken up by many others who have refined and streamlined their procedures, this also helps to explain why there are now basically three schools of reflexology.

1) The original Fitzgerald-Bowers school promoted by the Modern Institute of Reflexology,

2) The "Ingham Method," and

3) Other schools which incorporate Chinese acupressure points, among others.

Although there are "purists" who earn diplomas from the various reflexology schools around the world, most incorporate many different styles into their practice. As such, this book will neither distinguish, nor promote, one particular method. It will instead explain the basics commonly understood and used by most practitioners.

There has been a resurgence of interest in alternative healing techniques over the last few years, especially with the failure of modern medicine to combat most chronic illnesses such as cancer, diabetes heart diseases and respiratory conditions; with often the treatment is as bad as or worse than the cure.

Reflexology works. Fortunately for you, this book will explain how it does so (sort of), why it is so effective for some things, and how you can do it on yourself and on others.

Warnings

Reflexology therapy is not advisable for people who have the following conditions: deep vein thrombosis, thrombophlebitis, osteoarthritis, and cellulitis on the feet or legs, acute infection with a high fever, strokes or an unstable pregnancy. If you have a foot fracture, unhealed foot wound, or active gout in the foot, do not have reflexology.

Chapter 1: When Should You Use Reflexology?

Reflexology can be an enjoyable massage in itself. It is often used regularly to prevent the onset of disease, as well as to maintain optimum levels of physical and mental health. Many people have an opinion on reflexology, some people except it as a necessary and useful legitimate medical technique while others think of it as another sham or fad cure, but often their view on reflexology is gleamed from secondhand or third hand advise or information from someone who doesn't really know the facts to start with, much of the media anti-reflexology hype is propagated by those who have a vested interest in demoting it, such as the large drug companies and the orthodox or contemporary medical establishment who are always jealous of competition. As always with every branch of alternative medicine, there are those who make extravagant and unsubstantiated claims, but those who use and administer the therapies of reflexology and also those who have benefited, know the truth of the matter. My hope is after you have read this book you will be able to form your own balanced opinion on reflexology based on the real facts and be able asses its true value. I hope you will then decide to use it for your own and your associates' health benefits, whether you intend to use it privately or would like to make it a profession.

Most people use reflexology in conjunction with other treatments, a few resort to it in order to cure an ailment, however, as reflexology is painless, drugless, and doesn't involve surgery. Reflexology is used by millions of people of all walks of life in all parts of the world; it has been used to complement other treatments for such conditions as headaches, anxiety, nervous disorders, PMS, sinusitis, asthma, diabetes, eating disorders, obesity, kidney function penile dysfunction, cardiovascular issues and cancer treatments. But it is not used to diagnose or cure health issues or disorders on its own. You should not give up on conventional medicine – especially if you are already undergoing treatment for an existing condition, but use reflexology in conjunction with or as well as it, and in consultation with your doctor or healthcare advisor. Reflexology is also often used as a preventive measure because it is able to help relieve stress and unblock the various different cell communication pathways in the body.

Our bodies took millions of years to evolve, in order to do so; they needed to have their own self cure systems. Without these self-cure systems in place and working to optimum efficiency our species could not have survived. The unnatural external repair service provided by doctors has in terms of evolution, only been around for a very brief instant, but long enough to seriously disrupt our natural healing abilities. Reflexology helps our bodies own systems to do their job in a gentle, non-evasive way, with no side effects of health concerns.

The National Center for Complementary and Integrative Health (NCCIH) has found that reflexology has no side effects, whatsoever. This doesn't mean they think it works, mind you -- only that they find no harm in it, whatsoever. The British Complementary and Natural Healthcare Council (CNHC) concurs.

It is very important that you thoroughly understand that last paragraph. The American NCCIH and the British CNHC are government regulatory bodies which looks into and monitors alternative forms of medicine. Reflexology qualifies as an alternative form of medicine, a category it shares with acupuncture and other such forms of treatment.

These governmental organizations have looked into the claims of reflexology from a medical perspective, and have come up with very mixed reviews. Studies conducted by the National Cancer Institute, by the National Institutes of Health, and by others, have shown that while reflexology can indeed deliver on some of its promises, its other claims are rather dubious.

Reflexology can allegedly treat the following problems:

1) Anxiety
2) Arthritis
3) Asthma
4) Back pain
5) Depression
6) Diabetes (some types)
7) Digestive disorders
8) Fertility problems
9) Hormonal imbalances
10) Irritable Bowel Syndrome (IBS)
11) Migraines
12) Pregnancy issues
13) Preparation for labor
14) Relaxation
15) Respiratory conditions
16) Sinusitis
17) Sleep disorders
18) Sports injuries
19) Stress reduction
20) Toothaches

Some reflexologists make even more spectacular claims, which include cancer relief and others. This is not supported by the science, however, nor by other reflexologists.

It has been proven that reflexology can indeed reduce pain and stress in the same way that massage and taking a deep breath can – by relaxing the body. Many diseases are actually the result of stress and anxiety, which is why placebos work so well.

If you don't know what a placebo is, it's nothing more than a sugar pill. Doctors tell their patients that it is a wonder drug, and because most patients trust and believe in their doctors, they take the pill and feel better.

This doesn't mean that sugar is a medicine. All it means is that since the illness was in the mind, it is the mind that did the healing. Put another way: it was the patient's *belief* in the placebo's efficacy, not the sugar content, which cured the patient.

This does not mean, however, that reflexology's efficacy is all in the head. The health benefits of massage have long been established and is an accepted tenet in the medical field, after all.

That matter dealt with, modern medical science is a work in progress. This is evidenced by the fact that established medical theory and practice keep changing. What was yesterday's indisputable fact, is today an outdated theory.

In other words, more and more people are beginning to understand that their doctors don't know everything. Nor do they always have our best interests at heart. The pharmaceutical industry is far too close to many medical practitioners for comfort, while the commercial motive of many treatments (and reputations) leave much to be desired.

That aside, reflexology must never *ever* be used in lieu of conventional medicine, especially if you have a serious medical problem. Reflexology must only be used as an aid, not a replacement, for conventional medical treatment. If you are undergoing treatment for something, talk to your doctor first before undergoing a reflexology session.

With that in mind, reflexology is an effective treatment for relieving some forms of pain, especially headaches and migraine, anxiety, depression, sinus problems, stress, and many other ailments which will be covered in greater detail later.

As a form of massage, it has no side effects at all. It is therefore safe to do on yourself and on others. Just don't expect it to be a cure-all.

A few studies have been done to demonstrate the effectiveness of reflexology, one study in 2000 on the effect that reflexology had on cancer patients found that foot reflexology significantly reduced their symptoms of anxiety, and also helped with nausea and pain management. This is important because anxiety and stress can have a big effect on the way and time it takes for someone to recover and it can also hamper a person's ability to respond to other treatments. There are specific regions on the foot that will help change the entire energy flow throughout the body if stimulated properly.

The hand has various areas that can be touched and massaged to help the entire body relax. When someone's hands are tensed it can be a sign that your and possibly your whole body could be physically stressed. By using the reflex points in your hands, reflexologists release the trapped tension and let your entire body calm down. People often show they are stressed by having a closed or clenched hand with tense fingers. An open palm with loose, dangling fingers is a sign you are more relaxed. To demonstrate what they are doing while working on your hands a reflexologist will often show you a chart that depicts various regions they are using to stimulate or relax you on your own hand.

If you get frequent tension headaches or stress headaches, this can be a sign that your entire body is stressed. Your reflexologist may target the area of your head using various points in your Feet, hands or ears. Sometimes cortisol production and epinephrine can take over your normal system, in which case your sympathetic nervous system will dominate, making it extremely difficult for you to relax. Although it is less common, there are some reflexologist who now use **Face Reflexology Techniques** to target the head region_to help you calm down.

The stomach area is a very common point of focus in the treatment of anxiety with reflexology is the stomach area. Working to soothe this area will help calm down an overactive nervous system, known as a chakra (or energy system) that is located between your rib cage and navel system. The idea is to reduce that uncomfortable feeling in your stomach; some people with this condition have been known to suggest they feel like they have a knotted stomach or a lot of butterflies in their stomach. Reflexology will help to calm down these feelings in this area and relax you allowing healthy breathing and reduce the physical toll that stress has taken on your body.

Reflexology is sometimes mistaken for acupressure, but these two disciplines are completely separate – although some reflexologists do dabble in acupressure. The latter is based solely on Traditional Chinese Medicine (TCM) and works all over the body and the head, though it also stimulates acupoints on the hands and feet.

Reflexology is not just great at mitigating or getting rid of pain, but it is also effective at getting to the root cause of that pain. It is little wonder, then, that it has become one of the most popular forms of complementary medicine. The alternative is to use drugs, which can be very expensive, at best, or have negative side effects, at worst. It's also a lot cheaper than most conventional forms of treatment.

Chapter 2: How Reflexology Works

No one really knows. Different schools and practitioners have their own theory, which is another reason why reflexology is considered to be an alternative form of medicine. The accepted definition of Reflexology is that it is a gentle manipulation or the pressing on certain parts of the foot hands or ears to produce an effect elsewhere in the body.

Many practitioners of reflexology work on the theory that they manipulate the natural energy, life force or Qi to equalize and maintain the natural flows in the body's energy fields between cell and organs, these flows are the body's communication systems between the brain other cells and organs. The body uses several different pathways to send messages, some messages are sent by minute electrical pulses, other are sent using chemical compounds that are released as needed.

Many recent studies have revealed our bodies are negatively charged under "normal" circumstances, this negative charge can be changed to a positive charge by not being connected to the ground. All animals are almost always connected to the ground or grounded which keeps them negatively charged, but our modern human lifestyle has often removed us from our natural grounding by the wearing of synthetic footwear, the insulating of our homes with carpets and vinyl floor coverings, wearing clothing that produces a static positive charge, rubbing against synthetic materials and the influence of electrical wiring and electronic devices near the body. All of these can cause our systems to become positively charged until we become grounded so the charge dissipates. This change of the body from neutral or negative to positive can cause abnormalities within the system, often in the form of blockages or damage to the pathways causing stress and or pain as well as preventing natural and other types of healing. There is some suggestion this could be a major factor in many of the chronic illnesses that plague modern man especially cancers. Reflexology is very useful in helping the body to repair these blockages or abnormalities ensuring that the right signals or messages are sent and received by the cells they are supposed to.

Another communication system within our bodies are the chemical pathways using our blood, which also provides nutrients and oxygen to our cells and the lymphatic system which is largely the waste disposal system of our cells. Both these carry important chemical messages, usually in the form of enzymes, from cells to other parts of the body. These systems can be disrupted by trauma caused by accidents or even surgery as well as from chemicals that have been introduced into our system from our diet and also from electrical interference. The overeating of proteins has also been shown to have a dramatic effect on all the body's systems, when excess protein is broken down it forms a variety of disruptive compounds such as sugars, ammonia and uric acid. Our systems are also exposed to toxic preservatives, flavorings, colorings, fungicides and pesticides all of which pollute our systems; these are usually consumed along with processed simple carbohydrates that add to high blood sugar levels, adding more complications to an already stressed system. Apart from the many other problems that are caused by consuming these hazardous, unnatural, introduced chemicals, they can place a huge amount of stress on all of our delicate internal systems, causing inflammation, irritation and blockages which reduce the efficiency of the immune system and sometimes can cause varying degrees of pain. Reflexology can be used as a preventative strategy to strengthen the different systems, making them less likely to be affected by these hazards and also to assist the repair of these systems when they are stressed.

The other system that many different "Alternative Medicine Disciplines" as well as almost all "Cultural Based Medicine" such as Australian Aboriginal, Native American, Chinese, Indian and other Eastern types of Medicines use are the "Life Energy", "The Life Force", "Chi", "Qi", "The Hum or Buzz" or for those of us who remember the Star Wars movie where they described the energy as "The Force", these are concepts many westerners find hard to grasp or accept. They say that there is no scientific evidence for them, although they will tell you they accept such things as Luck, Bad Luck, Fate, Destiny, Divine Intervention and UFO's, things which are also in the category of "without substance or having any scientific evidence to prove they exist". Most people from Eastern or Asian, as well as from so called primitive cultures accept these ideas as basic fundamentals of life. This is an area that is difficult to describe and has to be taken on trust or faith, but if you refer to the previous chapter about placebo's efficiency in conventional medicine, it appears to me there is very little difference, it is a matter of having confidence in your Healthcare Professional and their ability to provide quality healthcare.

Reflexology is primarily used to stimulate the body to start repairing itself. Reflexologists use manipulation of the various points that they know relate to specific areas (as can be seen on the reflexology maps on the succeeding pages) to relieve any stress blockage or pain. When these areas are stimulated they send a message to the nervous system telling it to release chemicals such as endorphins that are the body's natural agents it uses to reduce stress and pain. As is to be expected the conservative medical community rejects these ideas outright, with the statement that there is a total lack of scientific evidence and it is contrary to the time proven form of medicine they use, which is largely a slash and burn approach to remove the symptoms so that the disease will cure itself, never mind the cause, medication (drugs) will cure and treat all.

There have been all manner of arguments and debates about the pros and con of reflexology, is it a treatment or merely a trick to extract money from the unwary. One interesting fact is there is a shortage of people who have undergone a full reflexology treatment by a qualified Reflexologist who claim it had no benefit for them personally. Where the opposite is true in that there are thousands of people all over the world who will testify to the positive effects they have personally experienced after undergoing reflexology, and millions of people who regularly opt for having reflexology sessions. Obviously, people would not be willing to spend their time and money if they found there was no benefit from undergoing these treatments.

Functional magnetic resonance imaging (fMRI) has proven that reflexology does indeed have an impact on certain organs. Pressing certain points on the feet has been found to increase blood flow to the kidneys and intestines, for example. What doctors still don't understand, however, is why it does so.

Imaging scans have also found that pressing different parts of the feet tends to light up receptors in the brain and baroreceptors (which are neurons) in the heart. Again, no one yet knows why this happens.

Lacking conclusive and scientifically verified answers, therefore, reflexologists resort to four major mainstream medical theories to explain how their system works:

1) Central Nervous System Adaptation Theory

This states that there is a relationship between the skin and organs through the nervous system, because the nervous system suffuses the entire body. As a result, you can't get hurt in one part of your body without having your entire body react to that pain. So even if you just prick your thumb with a needle, your whole body will reflectively jerk in response to that puncture wound.

This theory suggests that the central nervous system creates stronger links (to avoid being too technical) between different parts of the body. If you've ever bumped your elbow the right way, for example, then the tips of your fingers will go numb – a phenomenon known as the funny bone. Yet it was your elbow, not your fingers, that got hit, right? That's a "strong connection" between your elbows and fingers right there.

It is now understood that this is because of the ulnar nerve. This nerve let's your brain become aware of your fourth and fifth fingers, and lets you sense and control movement in your hand. Hit your elbow the right way so it bumps against (or squeezes) your ulnar nerve, and voila! There's that funny bone for you.

It has been suggested, therefore, that the central nervous system has a similar set up which directly connects certain points in the feet and hands with various organs in the body.

2) Gate Control Theory

This one's a bit more complicated and has to do with how the brain functions. Have you ever cut yourself, but didn't realize you did, till you saw the blood? Or have you ever been hungry, but didn't realize it, till you saw or smelled food? Well of course you have.

Discomfort is your body's way of telling you that there's a problem. Maybe you've been sitting down too long, or perhaps you haven't changed position in a while, so you are cramping up or a limb has fallen asleep. It could also be telling you that you need to eat or drink something.

Pain is the body's way of telling you that there's a serious problem – it could be a sickness, a burn, a cut, an open wound, or a hard bump. It is your body's way of telling you to look at and address the issue right away.

So how to explain being hungry or getting cut, but not realizing it?

Medical theorists suggest that although we have pain receptors all over our body, they're no good unless our brains register that pain or discomfort. If you get hurt, for example, and fall asleep, you don't feel the pain while you are sleeping. The cause of your pain hasn't gone away. It's just that your brain no longer registers the pain while you are asleep.

So this theory states that while the damage is in your body, the experience of pain is in your head. Since reflexology is a form of massage that relaxes people and improves their mood, the brain gets lulled into a state where it no longer registers the pain.

3) Vital Energy Theory

Also called the Yin and Yang Theory, this is based on Traditional Chinese Medicine (TCM). According to TCM, the body needs vital life energy, called chi, in order to function properly. Channels, called meridians, suffuse the entire body like veins – except that meridians flow in straight lines.

These meridians are what allows the chi to flow unimpeded to wherever it needs to get to. If these meridians are blocked, the chi cannot flow properly, resulting in lower energy and illness. This is also the theory behind how acupuncture works, by the way.

Reflexology doesn't make use of needles, however, nor does it stimulate other parts of the body as acupuncture does. It therefore suggests that every organ in the body has a corresponding acupoint in the hands and feet. By massaging the proper acupoints, the blocked meridians become opened, allowing chi to flow at optimum levels to wherever it needs to go.

4) Zone Theory

This states that every body part is represented in the hands and feet. Dr. Fitzgerald couldn't explain the exact hows and whys of the system, but he seemed to side with the Central Nervous System Adaptation Theory. Not knowing about TCM, he posited the idea that the body has several vertical zones which are inter-related. As such, the left foot affects the organs on the left side of the body, while the right foot controls the right side.

Chapter 3: The Essence of a Reflexology Session

In short, no one really knows exactly how or why reflexology works, but millions of people around the world swear by it. To make it simple, all you need to understand are five basic principles:

1) That the body is divided up into 10 longitudinal (head to feet) zones,

2) Each of these zones are further divided up into five zones – five on the left and five on the right,

3) Various points on the hands and feet correspond to different parts of the body,

4) A professional reflexologist can therefore sense any abnormality in the body by feeling the hands and feet, and

5) Massaging the appropriate points or zones stimulates blood flow to certain organs (which has been proven), nutrients (unproven), and stimulate the flow of energy (maybe) to maintain health (perhaps), mitigate pain (proven), and cure a host of ills (proven in some cases).

However, the pressure or zone points in the hands and feet are connected to the body's organs, they will be stimulated to ease pain or to strengthen areas of weakness in the system. Although reflexology can be considered to be a form of massage, no lotion or other form of lubricant is normally used throughout the session.

If you choose to have a session with a trained practitioner, it will begin with an intake procedure. This means that they will ask you questions about your health and lifestyle in order to better understand how to treat you.

Duly licensed practitioners are required by law (at least in America) to explain that reflexology *cannot* treat specific illnesses, and that it must not be used as a replacement for conventional medical treatment. You will also be required to sign a consent form to prove that you understand these points, as well as go release them from any liability claims.

Your Reflexologist is a trained professional so that you can expect that during your session with them, they will be polite and respectful of your individual needs and desires. They will stay focused, present and grounded with a calm manor and centered state of awareness, with your consultation as their only priority. In return you are expected to be honest and open and show them an equal measure of respect and common courtesy, in the same way that you would for any other professional who is helping you.

Reflexology like other forms of Alternative Medicine is open and upfront, your wellbeing is the main concern and with that theme in mind the idea is to make you feel comfortable and relaxed. Unlike conventional medical consultations, where the asking of questions is frowned upon and "heaven forbid", having an opinion on any part of your health is just not allowed or tolerated. When you are being treated by a Reflexologist you are encouraged to ask questions and give your opinions and observations on your condition. This not only helps your Reflexologist to determine their best approach to you and your therapy, but helps you to be relaxed and receptive as well as understanding what is happening and why. It is important to understand that reflexology is not to diagnose or treat any condition, but to help your body to relax and treat its self or sometimes to complement or improve other techniques that you may be using to treat or cure an ailment or disease.

Reflexology focuses on the entire pattern of reflexology therapy, not on any health condition or conditions you may have. For example, if you are having a reflexology session because you suffer from migraine headaches or another condition such as arthritis the whole session would still be the same regardless, starting at your toes and working down the foot or starting at the finger tips and working down the hand. Having one or two specific conditions as the reason for your consultation gives the reflexologist a reason to be a little more careful when working the area or areas corresponding to the condition you are seeking help to manage, but the reflexologist will still work carefully on all areas of the feet and hands with a gentle pressure because the reflexology theories are based on promoting the relaxation of the whole body and relieving the congestion or blockage of all nerve pathways throughout the body, as the body works as a whole unit not just as individual sections.

It should be understood that the reflexology therapist or Reflexologist stimulates the nervous system, this is to cause your body to respond or to do all the work of fixing or correcting problems, but it is not the therapist who does the fixing. When your Reflexologist finds an area of congestion or tightness that requires some work or remedies during your session they will apply the necessary proper techniques required to bring the whole body back into balance. If your therapist finds an area or areas of pain they will work on that area unlit they feel that harmony is restored to that area. Sometimes this will be accomplished in one session, but usually it will take several sessions to complete, the reason for this is because the body needs time to recover and recuperate, it is rare for quick fix methods to work. The goal of the reflexology session is not to try and fix any pain, it is to bring the whole body into balance and then the body will reduce the pain through its own natural methods.

A Reflexologist's job is to bring a sense of togetherness and overall balance to your body their purpose is not to diagnose or tell you about any congestion, tension or problematic area they observe that may suggest there is a problem or an abnormality. The reflexology session is to deal with stress and open up the nerve pathways with the main theory being that the body will nurture and repair itself when stress has been relieved or addressed. If a Reflexologist finds that your body is extremely stressed they would most likely refer you to an appropriate healthcare professional or medical team, but they will not give medical advice or diagnosis. This is not their field or job.

Although the focus will be on your hands and feet, some practitioners also pay attention to the ears. According to TCM, the ears are also a rich source of acupoints, so your treatment will also depend on the school your reflexologist received their training from.

There as stated earlier 3 different schools of reflexology so your Reflexologist may use slightly different techniques depending on which school they trained at, but they are all very similar. Because your therapist will work all points of your feet, hand and probably ears, they will cover or address all parts of the body, including the internal organs, glands muscles and muscle groups, bones and nerves, during a normal session. If you have an area that is of concern to you discuss this with your therapist and they will then be able to return to it at the end of your session to ensure it has been addressed.

Many people are a bit apprehensive about their first visit to a Reflexologist, but once you know the procedure, the application and the expected results, it makes it an easier decision to go ahead with having a consultation, the fact that there are no drugs involved no tests and no pain involved, makes the whole experience an enjoyable excursion.

Depending on the person there is a wide range of reactions people experience during a reflexology session. Many people experience a sense of relaxation and a sense of awareness of the area or areas connected to the specific points the therapist is working on. It is not unusual to feel a slight lightness or tingling sensation in the body, some people get a feeling of warmth, a sense of things opening up or energy starting to move when their therapist applies pressure or works on a specific area. It is also not unusual for people to sense a feeling or have a physical perception that there is energy flowing through parts or all of their body and that there is some form of internal communication taking place.

When you first arrive, you will be asked to remove your shoes and socks, and your feet will be washed with a moist cloth and/or soaked in a solution, after which they'll be dried. Reflexology is usually performed with you lying down on your back and with your feet sticking out over the edge of the bed. An alternative is with you reclining on a La-Z-Boy type of chair with your feet elevated.

The reflexologist will examine your feet, looking for any open wounds, rashes, sores, warts, bunions, and so forth. If you suffer from athlete's foot or other fungus that you did not disclose during your intake procedure, they may refuse to treat you. The same may apply if you have any similar conditions with your hands.

Some reflexologists will not treat diabetics or women in advanced stages of pregnancy, while others will. It is therefore best to shop around before settling on a practitioner, and to be as honest as you can during your intake procedure.

Sessions usually begin at your fingers and toes, before moving on to the rest of your hands and feet. The reflexologist may work to address one issue in the beginning, but during the session, they may detect other issues that need to be addressed.

Although reflexology can ease pain, that is not its primary goal. Reflexology aims to bring the body back into balance. The more it can do so, the less the body is likely to call out in pain by manifesting a condition like headaches, nausea, or fever, among others.

A session can therefore last anywhere from thirty minutes to an entire hour. Depending on the issue that needs to be dealt with, you may be asked to undergo three to six treatments for optimum results. These are usually done consecutively within the span of a week, but if your schedule won't allow it, let your practitioner know so they can tailor your sessions accordingly.

Depending on your state, city, and facility, treatments in America average about $30 for a half hour session, and around $55 for a full hour. Though lotion is not generally used, some practitioners like to apply aromatherapy oil, in which case, expect to see that reflected in the price.

Although a session is essentially a massage, and you may therefore expect to feel the physical sensations associated with one, some people become emotional during treatment. This is because emotions are not just fleeting things that occur in the mind.

All emotions, especially those that are repressed, manifest in our bodies in certain ways. This is why people who suffer a lot of stress eventually suffer from heart conditions, experience headaches, lack of sleep, or even panic attacks from out of the blue.

Your state of mind affects your body, your organs, and your focus. So just as prolonged stress can affect your body, so various emotions will have an effect, as well.

During reflexology, some of these deep seated emotions might come to the fore, especially if their causes are not addressed or ignored. Some people find themselves starting out a session in a calm and relaxed manner, only to devolve into fits of laughter or depression (sometimes both).

This is perfectly natural, however, and even expected. This phenomenon is called "releasing," which occurs when your body and certain internal organs relax enough to let suppressed emotions through. Reflexology doesn't just heal the body, in other words. It also has the power to release pent up emotions so you can let go of them.

Physical sensations may include:

1) Coughing
2) Disappearance of all pain and discomfort
3) Feeling as if all organs are hanging freely, not connected
4) Feeling cold or chilled
5) Feeling light-headed
6) Loose and relaxed muscles
7) Muscle contractions
8) Overwhelming desire to sleep
9) Perspiration of hands or feet
10) Sighing deeply
11) Thirst

Once a session ends, you will be asked to relax for a moment and not get up right away. Since it is common to feel thirsty after a treatment, you may be given some water to drink.

Once you leave, other symptoms sometimes occur. These can hit you hours or even days after a session, which include:

1) Better sleep
2) Emotional or psychological release
3) Flu-like symptoms
4) Frequent bowel movements, diarrhea (as toxins get eliminated)
5) Increased energy

6) Increased mucus
7) Kidney stones coming out with urine
8) More mobile joints
9) Nasal discharge
10) Relief from pain
11) Skin rashes, spots, or pimples (again due to the elimination of toxins)
12) Tiredness
13) Vaginal discharge

These are all normal reactions to a reflexology session and are no cause for alarm. Be sure to let your reflexologist know, however, so they can monitor your progress. At the risk of being too repetitive, also inform your GP, especially if you are undergoing treatment for something.

Sessions are also open to those without ailments as a form of tune-up in order to maintain health, balance, and focus.

Chapter 4: Applying Reflexology – Some Things to Bear in Mind

Since there are no side-effects with reflexology (a statement backed up doctors and medical researchers on the payroll of the American and British governments), it is also perfectly safe to do on yourself. You must have massaged your own hands and feet, at some point, so you know it is true.

There are 12 things you need to keep in mind, however, when you decide to perform a session, either on yourself or on another. They are:

1) Be Comfortable

Reflexology has to be done in a comfortable and relaxed setting. It must not be hurried or stressed, something that applies to both the practitioner, as well as to the one undergoing the treatment.

If you are, it's working on another person, have them lie on their backs with their feet dangling over the edge of the bed. An alternative is to have them get on a La-Z-Boy chair (or something similar) and have them recline comfortably on it with their feet up and easily accessible.

If you are working on yourself, you might want to sit up in a chair with a comfortable back. You don't want to slouch, or that'll hurt your back, but neither do you want to be too stiff. It is important that you find the right balance between maintaining a proper posture, while still being able to work on your feet.

2) Start with the Feet

When starting out, do so with the feet. This is how it is taught to students during formal lessons, because there's so much data on how parts of the feet affect the different organs and glands of the body. It is also easiest to work on, because it is also bigger than the hands.

When working on yourself, you can only use one hand, obviously; while working on your feet allows you to use both hands. It is also been found that stimulating the feet has a faster effect in mitigating pain, while working on the hands takes longer to see results.

Bear in mind, however, that the hands and feet are not mirror images of the other in reflexology. Since your heart is on the right side of your body, for example, then heart conditions are to be treated through your left hands and feet.

3) Commit to the Whole Treatment

You have to do the hands and feet, not just focus on one or the other. If you have a toothache, for example, it is tempting to just pinch your toes and leave it at that, but you have to go back to the four basic theories on how reflexology might (or might not) work.

Reflexology is an alternative form of treatment, and like most such methods, does not see the body as made up of distinct and independent parts. Reflexology sees the entire body as being made up of inter-dependent parts, rather, so you can't just focus on one body part to get rid of a particular ache or pain.

If you do have a toothache, it is not just your teeth telling you that you need to go to the dentist. Your teeth are connected to your gums, which are in your mouth, which are in your head, which are on your shoulders, etc. That pain can also be symptomatic of something else (like high blood pressure, for example), so you have to stimulate all organs by pressing all the pressure or zone points on the hands and feet.

4) Creams and Oils Are Usually Only for Massage

Which doesn't mean you can't use them for reflexology, as many do. If you are stressed and need a break, use the cream or the oil, by all means. But if you really want to address some problem (like a toothache), it is best to set those bottles aside.

Although you have to stimulate all the pressure points, there are specific ways to do so, which will be addressed later. Oils and creams make the skin too slippery, which can make it harder to target specific points.

There is also the temptation to just do a kind of gliding Swedish-like massage over the skin. While pleasurable to the one receiving the massage, however, such gliding motions ignores or ends up giving too little attention to the spots that need more pressure than others.

5) Massage Is Optional

Many professionals incorporate some type of massage into their sessions, so you can do so, too. If you choose to do this, you might want to start with a regular massage first, especially if you are going to use oil or lotion.

Once the massage portion is finished, be sure to wipe or wash the skin to get the cream off, then use the powder to absorb the excess. An alternative is to start with the session, then wipe the powder off if you want to use some type of cream.

A far better alternative is to learn some massage techniques that can be applied without having to use some sort of lubricant. Swedish massage is out of the question since it relies on rubbing motions. Shiatzu, which requires pressing acupoints, is ideal for such cases.

6) Use Talcum Powder

Baby powder works just as well, though if you are really desperate, so will baking soda (but only if you are in a pinch). Sprinkle this on the hands and feet to absorb the body oil and minimize slipping or gliding.

There is a method called thumb walking (again to be dealt with later), which will be hard to do without powder. If you really like the bells and frills, get a powder which comes with some nice and relaxing fragrance to lift the spirits.

Avoid strong, astringent scents which might encourage sneezing or be too stimulating. Reflexology must be done in a calm and relaxed setting. It should never be hurried or stressed.

7) Be Sensitive

If you are working on someone else, pay attention to how they react. A body builder might be able to take much greater pressure than a child, elderly person, or someone who's sick. It is even possible that due to an injury, certain spots might be more tender than others.

Although knowing which spots to pinpoint is important, it's also important to watch out for the person you are giving a session to. Some people try to hide their feelings (especially men who like to "suck it up"), but if you pay close attention to how they tense or hold their breath at some points, you'll know if you are going too far or not.

Your pressure should not be even, therefore. Some people can take more pressure on some parts of their hands and feet, but not as much on other parts. Also take note of the bones. Most people can take more pressure on the fleshy parts of their hands and feet, but less so on the bonier parts.

8) Some No-no's

Many reflexology schools caution students not to perform reflexology on those who have been in bed for 24 to 48 consecutive hours – the bed-ridden, in other words. Others caution against performing it on diabetics, while still others say the same about pregnant women.

In such cases, a massage might be more advisable. It should be made clear, however, that not all schools are in agreement on those aforementioned points.

What all do agree on, however, is sensitivity to the area to be treated. Do not perform a session on an open wound, a bruise, or suspicious rash. If said conditions appear on your own hands and feet and you still want to do it, then go right ahead. Do be careful if they appear on another person you intend to perform a session on, however.

9) How Long Should a Session Last?

Thirty minutes to an hour, though some go for 45 minutes. As you are obviously not a professional (or else why are you reading this?), it is best to do it for as long as you comfortably can. Or for as long as the person you are doing a session on can take it.

10) Dealing with Emotional Responses

This was already covered in Chapter 3, but just as a reminder – some people react emotionally to a reflexology session. If a novice like you is likely going to perform a session on someone you know, how you deal with it is up to you. Just know that an emotional reaction sometimes happens, so working on a perfect stranger is not advisable.

11) Don't Make Any Promises

At the risk of sounding repetitive – please remember that reflexology has not yet been proven to cure anything, at least as far as conventional medical science is concerned. It has been found to be effective at mitigating some forms of pain, but not all.

And while many swear that it has helped them with various conditions, many of those claims have not yet been subjected to scientific scrutiny. What this means for you is that you are in no position to tout it as a cure, nor forward yourself as the person to deliver that cure.

Creating high expectations in others, as well as giving yourself false hope, serves nothing. Try out the following exercises and see how well (or not) they work for you. Share your success stories (if any) by all means – but never make any promises about reflexology's ability (or yours) to actually heal anything. That is neither right nor proper.

In America, it also borders on being illegal – just look at what happened to Dr. Oz. And he's a certified health professional.

12) Drink Water After a Session

Since reflexology helps to purge toxins from the body, it is advisable to help those toxins on their way by drinking a glass of water after a session. Many who undergo a session feel thirsty when is it over, yet another sign that their bodies need to get rid of impurities. This is also why professionals provide water for their patients. Just be sure that it is just plain water and not something sweet or carbonated.

Since some people get chills after a full session, a hot cup of tea is sometimes offered. It all depends on how they (or you) feel after it's over. This is again natural, and not something to be alarmed about. While unsweetened tea, like green tea or Oolong is best, if you can't get your hands on them, then a little sugar is acceptable with regular tea.

Chapter 5: Understanding Foot Reflexology

You'll find the foot chart on the very next page, but before you get there, it might help to understand the basics of it so you don't panic. Once you understand how to look at the foot as a reflexologist would, it becomes easier to pinpoint what part of the foot corresponds to what part of the body. There is a very simple logic to the system, and once you understand it, the chart becomes easier to read.

The Foot Is a Model of the Entire Body

It is not at all complicated once you realize that the foot is considered to be the microcosm of the entire human body. This is why a reflexologist has you lie on your back (or partially reclined) with your toes pointing upward. In this position, you are presenting a three-dimensional model of yourself.

By working on the microcosm of your foot, the macrocosm that is the rest of your body is impacted. Your toes represent your head, so the rest of your feet represents the lower parts of your body in the same order. Your heels, therefore, represent your pelvic area, all the way to the knees, which are about as low as you can get in foot reflexology.

Head and Neck

The top, rounded, and fleshy part of your toes are manipulated to deal with problems which affect the head, and other things in the head region. Following this logic, the throat and neck are represented by the joints which connect the toes to the rest of the foot.

Spine

At the bottom of the toe joints, where they connect with the foot, is the spine. There's a lot more to this, of course, so you'll have to refer to the chart for further details.

Chest

The chest area is represented by the balls of the feet. If you put one foot on the other lap so you can see the bottom, fleshy part of it, you'll notice that the fleshiest balls of your feet are below your big toe and your smallest toe – an almost mirror image of your chest. Based on this, you develop a pretty good idea of where to find the points targeting the heart, solar plexus, and other parts in that general region.

Waist

The skinniest part of your feet (width-wise) are located about an inch or two above your heels, depending on the size and shape of your feet. Stomach ailments and other things to do with the waist area, are addressed here. Following reflexology's logic, things dealing with the groin, rectum, and so forth, are therefore below this region.

Diagram A: Right Foot Reflexology Chart Map

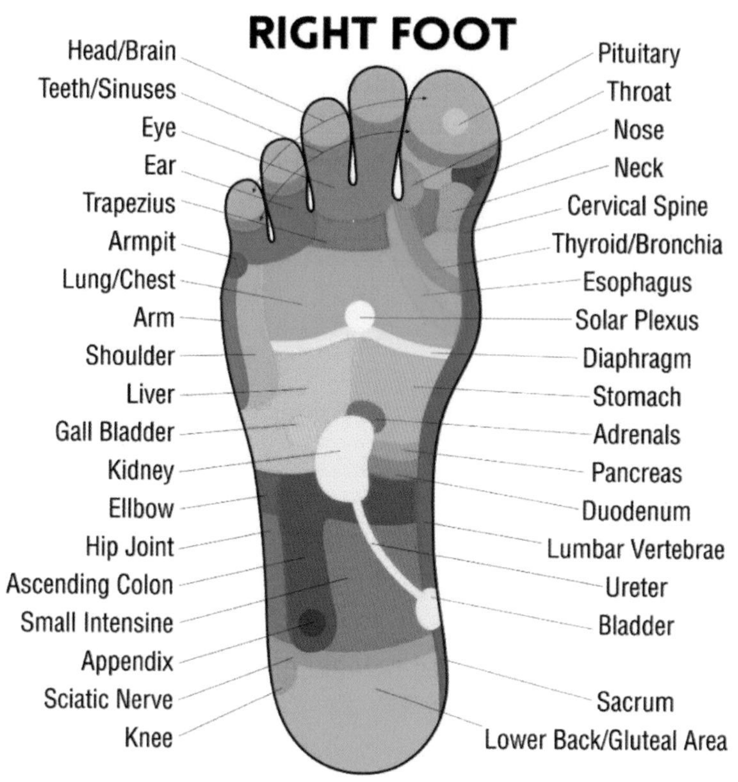

Diagram B: Left Foot Reflexology Chart Map

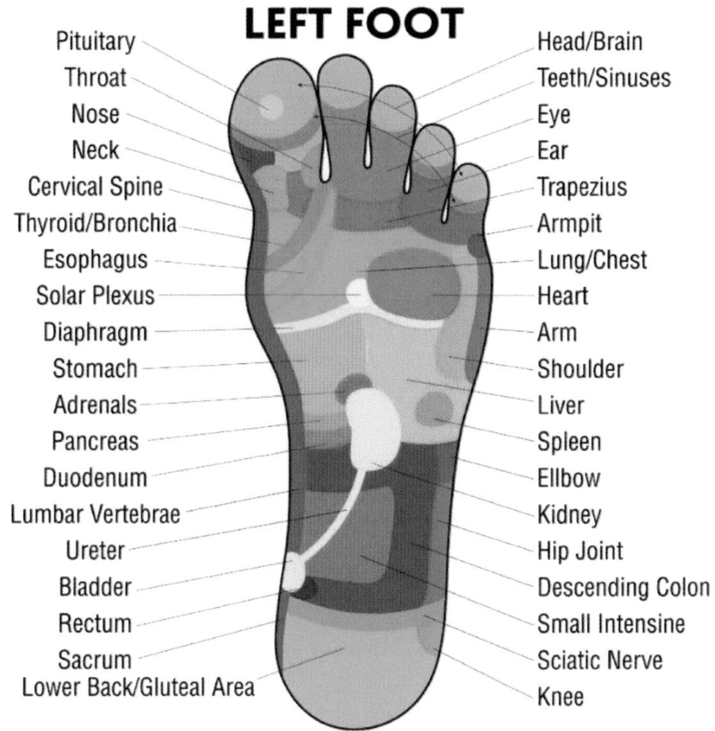

Now that you can see the chart, the logic becomes clearer. As it represents the bottom view of someone's feet, it should therefore be obvious that the foot on the left (your left) represents the other person's right foot, while the foot on the right represents *their* left.

Bear in mind again, however, that the feet are *not* mirror images of each other. Although the human body is symmetrical, its internal organs are not. The heart is located in the left side of the body, for example, so you'll only find its corresponding point in the left foot. The gallbladder, on the other hand, is only found in the right side of body, so you'll only find its corresponding point on the right foot.

Remember Dr. Fitzgerald's ten zones? That topic is a bit too advanced for the scope of this book, but remembering that it runs horizontally, from the head to the feet, helps to understand why the feet do not have symmetrical points. To make it simpler, just remember that the left foot is like a voodoo doll of the left side of the body, while the right foot serves the same purpose for the right side of the body.

To better help you locate certain points, such as the eyes and nose, consider how they appear on your face. Your nose is located between your eyes, so you'll find its point in the outer big toe (the part that faces away from the smaller toes). Using this reference, the points for the eyes can be found in one of the inner toes (the middle one, actually).

Chapter 6: The Five Methods of Reflexology Treatment

Although reflexology is not massage, most reflexologists include it as a sort of warm up in order to relax their patients. If the conventional medical establishment is correct that the only therapeutic benefits of reflexology lies in the relaxing, stress-busting aspect of it, then it can't hurt to do it on yourself or on another, now can it?

So start by holding one foot in both hands, such that your fingers cup the top half of the feet, while your thumbs do the actual massaging on the fleshy bottom. Begin with the toes first and move gently towards the rest of the foot till you end up at the heel.

Don't worry about the proper zone spots in the beginning, since this is only a massage to relax the patient. Since you can't touch any part of the bottom of the feet without impacting the organs, anyway, the session has already begun.

Be very careful to pay attention to the person's reaction as you do so. Are they wincing? If so, you are pressing too hard. Are they trying hard not to laugh? Oh, they're laughing already? Then you are probably putting too little pressure and are tickling them. Once you find the right pressure and the person is relaxed, you are ready to begin the actual session.

Reflexologists use five basic methods to stimulate the points, which are:

1) Thumb Walking

Thumb walking is the principle method used in reflexology. To better understand it, look at the upper joint of your thumb. Your sole focus should be on the area covered by your thumb nails. Or more specifically, on the pads opposite your thumb nails.

Your aim is to imitate the way a worm moves by using the tip of your thumb to pull the lower part forward, or by using the joint of your thumb to push the tip of your thumb forward. Start by pressing your thumb firmly against the skin, putting more pressure on the joint. Then you move the pressure to the tip of your thumb till it digs into the flesh. This is made easier with the help of talcum powder.

Be sure to cut your nails and keep them trimmed. If you have trouble exerting sufficient pressure on the foot, use your fingers to pull it forward against your thumb. For extra pressure, you might also want to lean forward with your upper body as you pull the foot toward you. This is especially good at mitigating the strain on your thumbs to reduce tiredness or soreness on your part.

2) Finger Walking

This is done on the top and sides of the feet, especially as they're bonier and are therefore more sensitive to pain. This requires more experience, but you might want to use it for the warm-up foot massage.

This method is similar to thumb walking, except that you use the upper tip of your index fingers. To reduce tiredness and keep the foot or hand balanced, be sure your thumbs follow your index fingers on the opposite side. Essentially, you are squeezing the hand and foot you are working on between your thumb and index finger.

If your index finger gets tired, replace it with your middle finger. Be sure to avoid the bones on the top of the feet, or you'll cause pain. You must only finger walk in the hollow between the bones.

3) Hook and Backup

Press your thumbs deeper into a point and keep them there for a few seconds longer. Then you ease the pressure and repeat the process on the exact same spot. This obviously requires more pressure on your part, so you might want to lean forward while pulling the foot toward you.

Again be careful, however, lest you hurt the other person. Push gently, at first, while paying careful attention to their reaction. Only press harder if they don't flinch or cry out. When doing hook and backup, special care must be done to avoid the bones. This technique is only used on the softer parts of the feet, so it must never be done on the toe joints.

4) Rotation on a Point

This is done on the balls of the feet. Press your thumbs beneath the balls of the big and little toes, technically known as the metatarsal heads. Use both hands to rotate the balls of the feet and the toes, first in one direction, then the next.

5) Press and Slide

Press the tip of your thumb against the foot above the heel. Now slide it up till it reaches the balls of the feet.

You want to maintain an even pressure from beginning to end. This is an effective way to target all organs. Again be careful to monitor the person's reaction to make sure you are not hurting them.

Use the Zones as a Guide

When you use these five techniques, pay attention to the zone you work on. Look at the toes. Now imagine that each toe has an imaginary line which runs all the way down to the heels. You want to work along these zones so that you can more effectively target the corresponding body part you need to reach.

Thumb walk from the side of the heel to the ball beneath the big toe. Return to the heel and thumb walk back up to the next toe, and so on till you reach the smallest one.

Chapter 7: Performing Foot Reflexology

Rotate the Toes

Grab the big toe and gently twist it from side to side. Work your way lower till you reach the joints. Some people have very sensitive toe joints, so be careful with the pressure of your squeeze. As a general rule of thumb, the thinner the skin above the bones, the more sensitive and prone to pain it is. Repeat this process with the other toes.

Stimulate the Toe Tips

Hold and stabilize one toe with one hand, then use the thumb of your other hand to press down gently. This isn't acupuncture, so don't worry about targeting the right spot. So long as you can cover the entire toe tip, you are good to go. Hold down for about ten seconds, and do the same for all the other toes.

Thumb Walk the Toes

Start at the base of each toe where it meets the foot. Thumb walk upwards to the tip of the big toe. Repeat this process with the other toes.

Thumb Walk the Balls of the Feet

The chest area stimulates the lungs, chest, arms, shoulders, esophagus, solar plexus, and esophagus, all of which are great for breathing, respiration, and energy. Start at the bottom of the ball beneath your big toe and do the same with the rest. You may then thumb walk vertically, starting from one side of the foot and making your way to the other side.

Finger Walk the Top of the Feet

Start at the gap between the big toe (also called the hallux) and the long toe (the one right next to it), and finger walk your way up to the ankle, taking care to stay between the bones. Repeat this process with the other gaps. Be sure to follow the index finger with the thumb, so that you are pinching the foot. The chest area, the lymphatic system, and the groin area are also found on the top of the foot to the ankle.

Ending the Session

Once the reflexology session is over, you can massage it again, followed by giving the foot and toes a gentle shake. Some also give the ankles a gentle twisting. Though different schools and practitioners have their own methods, this ending session is similar to the way masseurs give their clients a few quick (and gentle) karate chops on the limbs and back in order to "resettle" the internal organs and muscles.

Chapter 8: Understanding Hand Reflexology

Understanding how to read a hand reflexology chart is a little more complicated, but it generally follows the same logic as a foot chart. To get a really good grasp of it, you just have to pinpoint certain markers.

Head and Neck

The pads of the fingers represent the head and brain. The thumb tips, on the other hand, directly impact the pituitary gland (a pea-sized organ in the brain which controls the hormones responsible for growth, metabolism, and body mass).

You already know that the middle toes contain the points which correspond to the eyes, so it stands to reason that their corresponding hand points can be found in the middle fingers, as well. Using that same logic, the hand points for the nose can be found on the outer part of your thumb (the part which faces away from the other fingers) beside the fleshy, padded portion.

Since the points for the nose can be found in the thumbs, the rest of the neck must therefore fall below this point. The thumbs are therefore the marker for the central part of the body – head, neck, stomach, groin, etc.

Upper Body

Since the thumbs represent the central portion of the body, then it stands to reason that the further you get away from them, the closer you get to the sides of the body. With this as your guide, you should begin to understand how the rest of the body relates to the hands.

Below the pinky fingers, for example, are where you'll find those body parts and organs that can be found below the shoulders, such as the heart (in the left hand) and the appendix (on the right).

Solar Plexus

This is the sole exception to the layout. Although the solar plexus is in the middle of the body, its corresponding point on the hand is not beneath the thumbs. You'll find it beneath the balls of the middle finger, slightly above the center of the palms. Based on this marker, however, you then have an idea of where on the hand the other body parts can be found.

Lower Body

The points beneath the solar plexus marker correspond to the lower body. So to find the points which relate to the stomach and sexual organs, they must obviously be located below the solar plexus point.

Diagram C: Right Hand Reflexology Chart Map

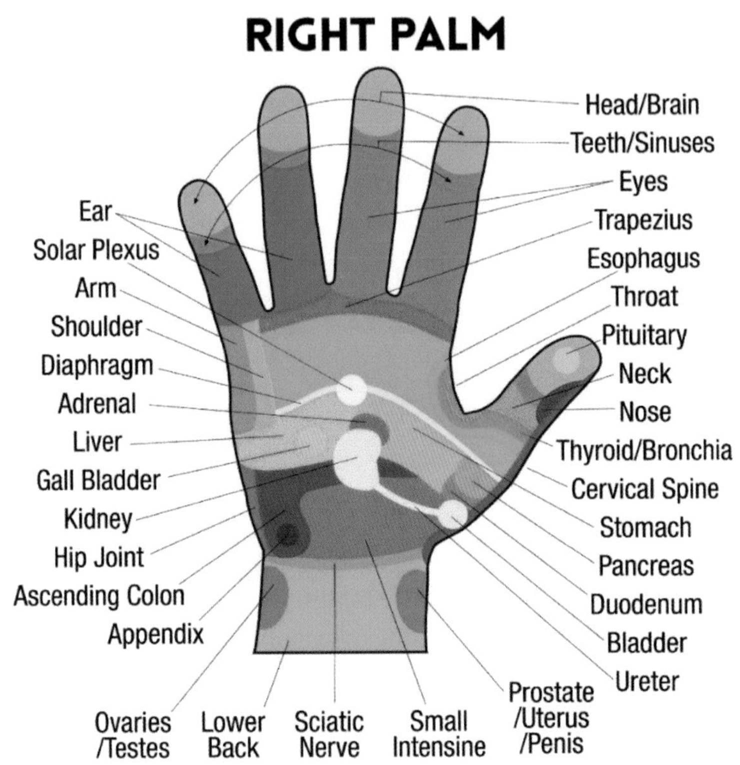

Diagram D: Left Hand Reflexology Chart Map

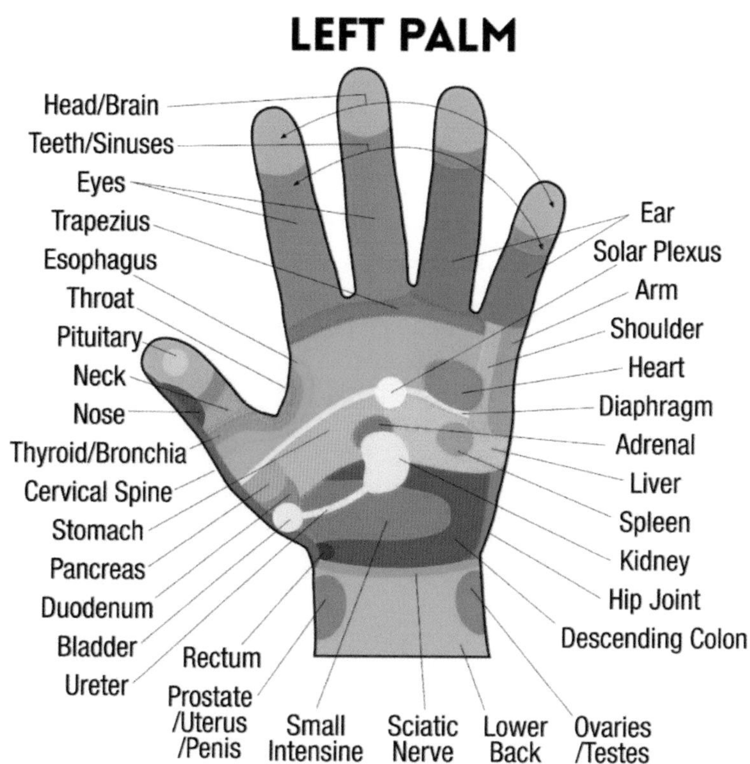

Some schools believe that hand reflexology is not as effective as foot reflexology, although those who make use of TCM disagree. Dr. Fitzgerald's books included many exercises for the hand, including gripping the teeth of a hair brush, as well as using clothes lines to squeeze the tips of the fingers. As such, those who use his techniques are also in disagreement regarding this point.

Whatever the case, all schools emphasize the need to stimulate both the hands and feet in order to complete a session and in order to achieve maximum results. If the foot cannot be massaged for some reason, perhaps because of an injury or fungal infection, then focusing on the hand will do. In such cases, however, it is believed that positive benefits take longer to manifest, so more sessions will be required.

Hand reflexology alone can also be performed in situations where taking off your shoes and socks might not be appropriate, such as in a formal office setting. You can use hand reflexology for relief from constipation, headaches, shoulder aches, and a number of other ailments which will be described later.

Chapter 9: Performing Hand Reflexology

The techniques for doing hand reflexology are not quite the same as with the feet. Your fingers must support the back of the palm, while your thumbs perform the massage. If you are working on someone else, hold their hands in both your own, working on one hand at a time. This will obviously be impossible when you are doing hand reflexology on yourself.

As with foot reflexology, divide the hands into five horizontal zones by imagining a line running from the fingers all the way down to the wrists. Starting and ending hand reflexology also involves a brief massage and perhaps a bit of a shaking, as well as the gentle twisting of the wrists.

The following are some generic hand exercises:

Thumb Walk the Palm

Thumb walk your way from the wrists to the balls of the fingers. Start with the thumb zones and make your way to the pinky zones. Now reverse that, working from the balls of the fingers and make your way back down to the wrist.

Thumb Walk up the Fingers

Starting at the base of the thumb, thumb walk your way to the tip. Do the same with the other fingers. Be careful to ease up on the pressure when you get to the joints, as these will be the more sensitive parts. Now make your way back to the thumb tip and work your way down.

Thumb Walk Horizontally

The palms can also be divided into three zones: (1) the balls beneath the fingers, (2) the middle of the palm, and (3) the two thick pads, one at the base of the thumb and the other at the base of the pinky. Thumb walk your way horizontally along these three zones.

Between the Knuckles

Turn the hand over so the back of the palm faces you. Although you can finger walk your way between the knuckles, thumb walking will also do if it is easier for you. Be careful, however, as this is the bonier part of the hand and can therefore be sensitive. Again, pay close attention to how the other person reacts. Now work in reverse, from the wrists back to the gap between the knuckles.

Twist the Fingers

Gently hold the thumb between your thumb and fingers. Now twist gently back and forth for about thirty seconds. Do the same with the fingers. Do not attempt to crack them.

Rotate the Fingers

Secure the person's hand by gently holding their wrist. Starting with the thumb, slowly rotate it in circles, first clockwise then counterclockwise. Again, do not try to pop the knuckles or finger joints.

Stimulate the Finger Tips

Use the index and middle finger of one hand to grab the back of the other person's thumb. With your thumb, press down on the other thumb for about ten seconds, as if holding a joy stick and pressing down on the button. Repeat this process with the other fingers. If the other person (or you) has long fingernails, it is alright to press down on the fingertip below the nails.

Squeezing the Fingers

If you are working on another, hold their wrist to steady their hand. With your other hand, gently pull the finger toward you, letting your hand slide down toward the tips of their fingers. Do not try to pop the knuckles, simply pull gently and slowly to activate the pressure points along the length of the fingers. If the talcum powder provides inadequate lubrication for this, use lotion.

Squeezing the Finger Tips

At the base of the fingernails, on either side, are more reflex points. Gently pinch the finger tips on both sides at the base of the nails, and squeeze slightly. There is a slight depression above the topmost finger joint, which is what you are after.

Thumb Walk the Wrist

Start at the bottom of the wrist, about two inches below the meaty part of the hand. Finger walk your way up toward the wrist. Start at the zone below the thumb and make your way to the other side. Now do it in the opposite order, starting at the top of the wrist and working your way down in the direction of the rest of your arm.

Rotate the Wrist

Hold the person's arm above their wrist. With your other hand, gently rotate the entire hand first in a clockwise manner, then reverse.

Chapter 10: Seven Do-It-Yourself Techniques for Various Ailments

The exercises in the previous chapters feel great, if you are the one receiving it that is. They're very basic exercises that can be used to promote health and well-being on their own as part of a regular tune-up. For a more effective tune-up, however, get yourself to a professional.

For more specific remedies, however, you might want to try the following remedies:

1) To Relieve Headaches

The foot is where you want to focus on for this. You can cross your legs in full lotus so you can work on both feet simultaneously, but it is best to work on one foot at a time. Using your thumb, rub the bottom of your big toe in a circular fashion, which will relax your neck.

Next, put some pressure on the upper part of your toes, as they correspond with the head. You should also massage the soft pads of your fingertips, as these also correspond to the head and brain.

2) To Deal with Sleep Problems

Remember how the fleshy part of the thumb affects the pituitary gland? This is the point you need to target if you have difficulty sleeping. Find the center of your thumb pad and give it a good squeeze with the thumb tip of your other hand. Next, squeeze the sides of your thumb at the points just above the joints, on either side of the base of your thumbnail. Do the same thing for your big toes.

Taking care to avoid caffeine and other stimulates before going to bed also helps, by the way. You might also want to avoid the glare of a TV, computer monitor, or cellphone, as the presence of light stimulates alertness and can interfere with deep sleep.

Studies have found that you can get a good night's sleep every night by working on your relaxation responses; reflexology has been shown to be very helpful for improving your sleep quality. To do your own reflexology for improving your sleeping, on your left foot, work your right thumb across the diaphragm line, from the inside to the outside edge. While you are doing this try to rock your toes back and forth across your left thumb and edge your right thumb along your diaphragm line each time you bend your toes over.

3) To Mitigate Stress

The head zones are covered by the soft padding of your toes, while the neck is in the fleshy bit of your outer big toes. Since stress usually manifests as tension in these areas, you want to squeeze their corresponding zones on your toes.

Another technique is to place your thumb in the middle of your inner wrist with your palm facing you. Place your index, middle, and ring finger on the outer wrist directly opposite. Now move your thumb and opposing fingers up and down so they roll the skin of your wrist from side to side. Doing so relaxes the sciatic nerve, the largest one in the body.

4) For Colds, Sinus, and Flu

Your sinus zones are in your middle finger, just above the topmost joint and below the fleshier bit on top. Your nose is represented by the fleshy, outer part of your thumb, while your throat lies in the fleshy bit below the index fingers just above the "V" it makes with the thumb. These are the points you need to stimulate to get rid of colds and flu. Find their corresponding points in your toes, as well.

5) For Asthma and Bronchitis

The lungs are targeted by pressing against the balls of the feet, about an inch below the toes. For the hands, target the soft padding at the base of your fingers. Turn your hand over. Press down on the gaps between, and a little below, the knuckles.

6) For Digestion Relief

Take a tennis ball, or similarly sized ball. If your hands are small, a golf ball will do, or something like it. One exercise involves locking your fingers together and squeezing the ball as hard as you can, which stimulates the digestive tract. You can also roll the ball between your palms as if you are shaping the ball, but put some pressure into it.

7) Back Pain

The spinal zone for the hands starts on the outer thumb just below the middle joint, and extends all the way to the wrist. Start at the wrist and thumb walk your way up the outer thumb till you reach the middle joint of the thumb. You can also put a bit of lotion on the spot so you can press and slide your way from the wrist to the thumb joint.

On your feet, the spinal joint stretches from the outer part of your big toes below the middle joint, all the way to the heel, ending just above the heel bone. Thumb walk from the heel all the way to the toe joint, and use cream or lotion to press and slide your way up.

Chapter 11: Reflexology for Weight Loss

Today's eating habits, the types of foods and lifestyles we enjoy are often not conducive to maintaining a healthy balance within our body's, many people now finding themselves in the difficult position of being overweight and not being able to lose the extra pounds. There are a multitude of diets and weight loss programs advertised in most social mediums, they all promise you will lose that weight and become lean and sexy, but without the right support it is often very difficult to stick to your chosen weight loss program. What is required is a practical method to reduce your weight down or back to your preferred or optimum size with the least stress possible, a method that does not involve harsh diets or strenuous exercise, but will give the desired results. Reflexology has given many people an edge that allows them to overcome temptation and remain on their chosen weight loss program.

Although Reflexology by itself will not cause you to lose any weight, what reflexology is able to do is by stimulating the correct points on the feet, hands and ears, it is possible to trigger responses in the body that will reduce hunger, stop cravings and also burn up the food you consume so it is not turned into fat. Reflexology is also useful in raising people's self-esteem, helping to cope with anxiety and depression which are often leading causes of people being overweight.

By having a suitable diet that is compatible with your body type, lifestyle and exercise level coupled with regular reflexology sessions to keep your body's systems on track and tuned to weight loss, as well helping to attain a harmonious and positive outlook, you have a very good chance of finding a pleasurable way to lose weight. (Most people on a regimen to lose weight that they dislike are doomed to fail, simply because is not enjoyable).

To lose weight with the aid of reflexology you can do it yourself with a friend or seek a professional to help you. The areas that need to be worked are the points that correspond to your spleen, stimulation of the spleen will help to reduce hunger. You are digestive organs, stomach, gallbladder and pancreas, stimulating these organs helps to improve your digestion. Another area that will benefit from being stimulated to control your eating habits are your endocrine glands, by stimulating them they will promote the secretion of hormones that can help control; your appetite, the thyroid and adrenals will help to balance your emotional and physiological stress and also help to motivate or make you feel more likely to want to do some exercise.

Self-Administered Foot Reflexology for Weight Loss

First refer to your foot chart and find the exact location of the points you wish to stimulate. For best results your weight loss reflex points should be worked at least for 5 minutes each day.

It is important that you feel comfortable and as relaxed as possible in all reflexology sessions. Find the most comfortable position sitting or lying down, some people may find it difficult at first to be comfortable, especially if over weigh. One way of becoming comfortable and relaxed is to use a flotation devise such as a water ring and do your session in a pool or in the sea. Being in the water allows you to be in effect weightless and it is easier to become comfortable and reach or place your foot in a comfortable position where you can work on it. Although it is preferable for your foot and hands to be dry if possible. The reflexology techniques will still work with water, as water does not cause the skin to become slippery. Some people may find that it is impracticable for them to try reflexology on their own feet for a variety of reasons so they should try the reflex points on their hands, by using one had to stimulate the other. (See the directions for doing this below.)

Support your left foot with your right hand and use your left thumb to work the spleen point. On the chart it is the oblong area indicated on the outside edge of your foot between your diaphragm line and your waistline. When you stimulate the spleen it has the effect of reducing the feeling of hunger.

In order to work on your stomach and pancreas reflex points, find a comfortable position where you can cradle your left foot with your right hand and using your left thumb, press each point. On the chart your stomach point is on the inside arch of your foot, just under the ball of your sole and your pancreas point is in the center of the inside arch of your foot. When you reach the outside limit of the reflex area, change your hands around so you are working the reflex points back in the opposite direction, the stimulation of these points will help to improve your digestion.

To stimulate your gall bladder, find the reflex point which is a small point located in the larger liver reflex area on your right foot, just below the ball of your sole, toward the outside of your foot. The gall bladder stores a digestive liquid called bile, this is continually secreted by your liver, its main function is to emulsify fats in your food that can then be used as energy in the body, this is conducive to weight loss and improves digestion.

Balancing your hormone secretion can help you over the cravings for those foods that are mainly sugars and help to feel inclined to want foods that are more appropriate as well as helping to balance your emotional and physiological stress. Your endocrine glands are responsible for your response to stress, applying pressure to the reflex points for your thyroid (at the base of your big toe), pituitary gland (in the center of the bottom of your big toe) and your adrenals (between your waistline and your diaphragm line) will help to address stress issues and can also help you feel motivated to exercise. The less stress you feel emotionally and the less stress you have in your body the better chance you have to stay on your diet. A tip for getting rid of that sweet tooth craving is to rinse your mouth with a glass of water that has a teaspoon of baking soda dissolved in it, this detunes your taste buds and with your reflexology stimulation, gives you a good chance of beating the need for extra munches.

Self-Administered Hand Reflexology for Weight Loss

For many or many people it is not practicable to use the reflex points on their feet, so it is fortunate the hands also provide key reflex points to facilitate weight loss. Using the hand is also very useful when you are on the go or unable to remove your shoes.

It is best to refer to the reflexology hand chart for the exact areas where you will find the reflex points. In general, the reflex points on your hands are located in a much smaller area than those on the feet and require a much firmer pressure, so press deeply, using a single finger or your thumb to apply the pressure, but not so as to cause or feel pain, it is also necessary to hold the pressure for longer than you would on your feet. The contact on the skin should be maintained as your finger creeps over the reflex point (s) in minute stages.

The reflex point for the spleen is below your little finger on your left hand. The reflex point for your digestive organs is below the lung and breast area on both hands. The gall bladder reflex point is the pad under the little finger on your right hand, and the endocrine glands reflex points are at the middle and base of your thumbs on both hands.

Chapter 12: Reflexology for Infertility and During Pregnancy

Reflexology to help cure infertility

In the United Kingdom reflexology is becoming a popular method for helping couples conceive. There are some points on the foot and hands that are associated with a woman's egg production, fallopian tubes and ovaries, by manipulating these areas reflexologists have had a lot of success in helping women to conceive as this helps to correct the imbalances which can hamper pregnancy, including unblock energy pathways in the body and so help the body to regain its natural balance and heal itself.

Reflexology has been shown to help couples with fertility problems by promoting blood circulation around the body, strengthening the immune system, balancing the hormone production necessary for conception to occur and promoting good strong health and vitality in the reproductive organs.

In order to prepare to conceive, time is need for the body to adjust especially if you have had problems conceiving in the past. Three months is about the right amount of time it will take for couples to become ready, because takes this long to produce healthy sperm and 1 month for a healthy egg. It would be ideal for both the male & female partners to have reflexology sessions or treatments to give the best chances of fertilization, this is especially true if no explanation or reason for the infertility is unknown.

A couple learning reflexology techniques to mutually stimulate each other is a winning formula that many couples have tried and succeeded with when trying to conceive, it can also strengthen their relationship and bring harmony into their lives.

For those couples who have chosen to have IVF, Reflexology can be used to help reduce the stress and emotional unease and help prepare the body physically.

Reflexology is now one of the most popular complementary therapies used by women during their maternity, because it helps to improve general well-being and vitality. It also induces a deep state of relaxation, allowing the female body to adjust to the many major changes which are taking place. Reflexology has been shown to help to ease or prevent many of the discomforts and ailments which are commonly associated with pregnancy. Long standing trials in the UK have found that those receiving regular treatments of reflexology during their pregnancy tend to deliver closer to term and have shorter labors.

Some of the many complaints that many women suffer from during their pregnancy and after, that can be relieved with the use of reflexology are:

Morning sickness, reduce and normalize high blood pressure, normalize low blood pressure, Oedema and reducing swelling in feet and ankles, nausea and headaches, pain and discomfort, backache, stress and anxiety, Improved sleep quality, digestive problems such as constipation and the relief or prevention of heartburn, adjusting to the demands of coping with a new baby, coping with interrupted sleep and fatigue, decreased energy levels, maintaining or increasing milk supply, support as your menstrual cycle returns to normal, re-balance the body and stabilizing body weight and the prevention of post-natal depression.

Most Reflexologists will not treat women in the first 13 weeks of their pregnancy because of the chance of inducing a miscarriage, also most professional places will NOT do foot reflexology on women before they are 37 weeks because of the labor triggers so I recommend that you take extreme care with doing any reflexology or massage while pregnant it is better to get a professional to do it for you and treat yourself.

Having said that the following are methods to induce and help during labor:

Apply firm pressure to the center of the thumb for about 3 to 4 minutes and then change to the other thumb and do the same. Keep the pressure on for 3 to 4 minutes. This method will help to induces uterine contractions. It stimulates the pituitary gland, which releases oxytocin, the hormone that induces labor.

There is a pressure point on the insides of the ankles, an inch or two above the foot. Gently work around until you find a tender spot and then apply pressure using your fingertips, keep applying the pressure until there is a contraction. Stop applying the pressure to the ankle as soon as you feel a contraction beginning. When a contraction has completed its cycle, begin to apply the pressure again.

Make sure you are in a comfortable position and using your fingers, apply pressure to the space about a finger width between the big and second toes. Continue with the pressure points in 15-minute intervals until contractions begin.

There is a spot or point on the arch of your foot, in front of your ankle. Gently feel around with your fingertips until you find it, it will be quite tender or sensitive, press this spot gently increasing the pressure until you feel some relief. This point helps in dealing with pain.

Some of the positive benefits of Reflexology during pregnancy are that it can help to oxygenate the mother's blood there by oxygenating and improving the blood flow in turn helping the uterus and the baby's placenta. It can also dramatically reduce any stress levels for the mother and baby, as well as helping to carry the baby to its full term.

Many women who are post-term in their pregnancy find it difficult at times to relax, when your baby is nearing the time it is due reflexology therapists use a method called labor priming, this is where specific reflex points are strongly stimulated to purposely create a boost of energy to encourage the onset of labor contractions. Most women who are post-term respond well to this therapy, with often one or two sessions being necessary, with the result of a quicker and easier delivery for both the mother and baby.

Your Health professional and Reflexologist are the best people to determine the suitability of treatment, but there are some conditions where it is universally recognized that reflexology should be avoided altogether during pregnancy and these include:

Pre-term labor (less than 37 weeks pregnant), Placenta Previa (low lying afterbirth) if grade ii or iii and 32 weeks or more, Hydro amnions if 32 weeks or more.

Chapter 13: Reflexology for Anxiety Disorders

Reflexology is often used for anxiety disorders and stress, because of its calming effect and because it does not use any medications to cloud an already stressed situation. Reflexologist's use it to supplement or add to an existing treatment of people who are struggling with anxiety and or stress. Often it is more effective than some of the very dangerous and addictive drugs that have been used to treat these types of conditions. If you have high levels of stress and anxiety, reflexology may be able to help you calm down and learn to control your anxiety symptoms. Most people go to a professional reflexologist for an initial consultation; this allows them and their health advisors to gauge their reactions and to see whether they respond to this type of alternative therapy.

Reflexology has been shown to be beneficial in helping with the restoration of the body's natural energy flows so they can be maintained at the right balance of both physical and mental functioning, there by promoting relaxation. One of the most common uses for this type of therapy is to help treat stress and anxiety. Reflexology has been found to help increase blood flow to the extremities, slow down heart rate, and decrease blood pressure. Because reflexology therapy is soft and has minimal pressure, it feels soothing to the patient. One of the extremely great things with this type of therapy is it is accomplished without any drugs or medication, just a trained professional.

Although it has been shown that it is not possible to have any negative side effects with reflexology, for most anxiety problems it is best at least in the beginning to seek the help of a trained professional to get the best results. Because of the nature of most anxiety problems and the way reflexology works it is normal to see results over a number of sessions. Once you have begun a series of treatments, although you may not be able to see a reflexologist every day to receive reflexology treatments, there are things that you can do in between treatment sessions to help keep anxiety at a minimum. Some people use hand reflexology on themselves to help control stress symptoms in between sessions with their reflexologist.

Usually a professional reflexologist will explain exactly what they are doing when they treat you and why they are doing what they do. They will also advise you on any self-treatments you can use between visits. Some of the areas they will stimulate to try and relieve your symptoms of anxiety are: They will also explain that they are not there to cure you, but to assist your body to overcome the problems that you have. In essence they are showing you and your body the way to heal itself.

The stimulation of the Adrenal glands, when experiencing anxiety, especially in heavy cases of anxiety your adrenal glands will be very sensitive. Often for some reason they have been kicked into overdrive and are overproducing epinephrine, this will keep your entire body on edge and alert. When these are overstimulated, you need to take the time to calm them down so that you can successfully function in society. Reflexology is ideally suited to helping you to relax.

Our brains are extremely complicated as everyone knows and are also very delicate; often anxiety is caused through over reaction to stimulants both physical and mental. Although some forms of massage will increase brain function, reflexology is tailored to calming our systems and opening pathways to drain away nervous energy allowing us to relax. If you are experiencing rapid thinking and are finding it difficult to calm yourself down, this therapy may gradually help. By becoming more physically relaxed, it opens the door for increased mental relaxation and often allows a better sleep.

Our Gut is an area that is now being recognized as playing an important part in our emotional wellbeing and it is now believed that a lot of stress and anxiety is linked to it especially with conditions such as irritable bowel syndrome (IBS) or other colon issues, reflexology treatment has long been associated with helping to provide relief for this type of ailment. Often there are cases where anxiety can have implications on the digestive system and colon, if your stress and anxiety is linked to any eating disorder.

Sleeping Disorders are often linked to the Pineal gland, especially if you are having difficulties falling asleep night due to your symptoms of anxiety. Reflexology helps to control the cycle of waking up and falling asleep, by changing your rhythm cycles and helping to reset natural functioning and aiding in falling asleep and waking up at good times.

The Pituitary gland is implicated in stress and anxiety as well as the body increases the production of stress hormones, it interferes in the normal natural functioning of the pituitary. When the stress levels begin to return to normal because the body starts to relax and emotional issues are addressed the pituitary helps promote normal hormonal activity and homeostatic functioning.

To boost energy and a relaxation aid by stimulating the adrenal gland

Find the point that lies between your middle and index fingers just below the thumb (see the hand chart). Gently press the thumb onto the reflex point of your free hand and apply a light pressure. Slowly curl up then straighten your fingers, a bit like making a fist and repeat this 10 to 12 times the do the same with the other hand.

To keep your hormones in good order by stimulating the pituitary and endocrine glands

Place one thumbnail in the center of the other thumbnail and push it in slightly (not to cause pain) and hold it there for about 30 seconds repeat with the opposite thumb and do this several times a day.

To reduce emotional stress and aid with sleeping

Sit with you back supported (it should be straight) and without any foot wear, gently place one foot so it rests on the other knee. Try to place it so you can see the base of the foot. Look for the point that lies at the base of the balls of your foot (see the foot chart), slightly above the arch of the foot. Place your thumb at the base right in the center and then apply a steady pressure until you feel a slight pain and massage the point a little, then repeat with the other foot.

To relieve feelings of anxiety and panic

Grip your right index finger with your left hand and squeeze it gently. Keep holding your finger until you can feel your pulse or heartbeat. Do this with all your fingers the change hands and do it with the other fingers.

Chapter 14: Reflexology for Back Pain

It is a good idea to prepare your legs and feet before you state your reflexology session, to do this, use gentle but firm pressure to massage your calves, ankles, soles of your feet, and toes and then flex your foot forward and backward, and then rotate your foot to loosen up your ankle.

For General Back Pain

Massage the lower arch-edge of your foot for 5-10 minutes. This area corresponds to your lumbar area and will help relieve general back pain.

Lower Back Pain

Lower back pain is best treated by applying pressure to all the reflex points on the soles of your feet, the entire area around your heel an ankle, as well as the inner edge of each foot.

The spine is treated by applying pressure to the areas along the inside edges of your feet.

Upper Back Pain

Upper back pain is treated by applying pressure to the reflex points for your shoulders and upper back, which are represented on the soles and tops of your feet just beneath the base of your toes. Use your thumb to apply pressure to the area just beneath the base of your toes, first on the sole of your foot and then on the top of your foot. On the soles of your feet there is a lot of flesh so you can also press your knuckles deeply into those reflex points. On the tops of your feet, use a lighter touch for the same reflex points because that area is more bony and sensitive.

The reflex points for the spine follow the line of the inside edge of your foot; these reflex points are not on the sole of your foot.

Sit with you back supported (it should be straight) and without any foot wear, gently place your right foot so it rests on the left knee, with your right foot supported, use your right thumb to work all of the spine reflexes that are located along the inside edge of your foot, from the tip of your big toe all the way to your ankle. Start with your big toe press your thumb firmly into the skin and move slowly along the whole length of your foot so you are sure to press every reflex spot.

To work on your Sciatic Nerve

Sciatica causes searing pain down the leg because the nerves are compressed, which can be triggered by a number of factors.

The reflex points for the sciatic nerve are found just behind your ankle bone and continue up in a straight line for about 4" or 10 cm. Working the sciatic nerve reflex points every day for a few minutes is a great way to prevent a painful case of sciatica and improve the blood supply to this area. His is best done by using your index finger and thumb to press gently on the area. Move your finger and thumb back and forth, bringing them together and then sliding them apart.

Using Hand Reflexology

Sometimes it is more convenient to use hand reflexology, some people suggest that it is not as effective as using foot reflexology, but I feel it is a matter of personal choice and preference, often if the feet are injured or infected they cannot be used and people still get good results.

The Spine

The reflex points for your spine are located along the outside edge of your palm, use your thumb to apply pressure and the switch hands.

Shoulders and Upper Back

The reflex points for your upper back are located just beneath your little and ring finger on the top of your hand, they are worked by applying pressure to the area, the left hand corresponds to left side and right to right side On the palm of your hand, the area for your shoulders is located just beneath your pointer and middle fingers. There is also a reflex point for the upper back on your palm just below the base of your thumb, on the outside of your hand.

Chapter 15: Reflexology for Addiction

Although Reflexology is not a cure for addiction or a substitute for therapy, it is however now widely accepted and is becoming increasingly popular at treatment centers around the world as an effective complement to any other type of therapy including a holistic addiction treatment.

Reflexology improves blood circulation, which promotes the healthy flow of oxygen and nutrients to the tissues. It is beneficial when used in the recovery of substance abuse and addiction, because it helps remove toxins in the blood, which results in fewer cravings and reduces symptoms of withdrawal. People using reflexology often report an instant feeling of relaxation, reduction of anxiety, increased energy and an overall sense of wellbeing after the first session, which makes it easy for them to engage in further sessions.

A popular theory of why some people form addiction suggests that people become dependent on substances like alcohol or drugs because they come to associate them with good feelings. Specific substances in the bloodstream have now been identified, such as dopamine and serotonin, which appear to be related to causing these feelings.

Everyone feels this process of association and we all tend to be drawn toward things that make us feel good. When you sense or even just think about something that has made you feel good in the past, such a lover or a favorite food, our bodies are programed to want or crave for another dose of the dopamine that goes along with it. Therefore, people are drawn toward that stimulus.

During a session to help relieve the feelings associated with addition a Reflexologist will work on stimulating the hypothalamus, pineal, and pituitary glands to release more Serotonin, Melatonin and Dopamine, which are known as the happy hormones or mood boosters, because they provide the feeling of pleasure, they make us feel content, happy and sociable. The reverse can happen when these hormones are at low levels or lacking, they can contribute to a person's feelings of irritability and depression can contribute to irritability and depression.

Studies have found that in the early stages of withdrawal from alcohol or drugs, including tobacco have significantly reduced levels of dopamine in their bloodstream. This causes negative feelings and increases the desire or craving for the substance they are giving up. Reflexology can help to replace that empty feeling until their bodies readjust and they begin to enjoy other activities and stimuli in place of the substance they were addicted to.

During or shortly after a reflexology session for withdrawing from any substance (and occasionally with just normal reflexology sessions) some side effects may occur as a result of toxins being emitted from the body. Any negative side effects which occur are not expected to last any longer than 24 hours. Such results may occur in someone who first experiences reflexology, but are unlikely to occur again and are only the result of the positive changes being made in the body.

To help with giving up smoking it is most common for each session to begin with the stimulation of the points on the foot linked to the solar plexus, which should help you relax. Once the person is relaxed, then the reflex areas for the lungs are stimulation along with areas for the diaphragm and heart, as well as the adrenal, pineal, pituitary and thyroid glands and those reflex points that relate to the function and health of the brain. The stimulation of these areas helps to ease the body's craving for nicotine. It is often necessary to have sessions of 15 to 20 minutes every second day or at least twice weekly as well as whenever the urge to smoke becomes hard to resist.

Chapter 16: Understanding the Different Styles of Reflexology

The Main Differences between the Chinese and Western Styles of Reflexology

The question that is often asked is what is the difference, if any between the Chinese and Western versions of Reflexology? They are very similar, but they do have some fundamental differences. The most notable differences are the intensity of the pressure applied while stimulating the reflex points and that the position of some of the reflex points is different.

In Western reflexology the amount of pressure applied or the intensity of the massage in never so hard as to cause discomfort or pain, with it usually being a pleasurable sensation and kept inside the "pleasure zone", but not so light as to tickle. The amount of pressure used on the hands is often a little greater than the foot, because the points on the hands are smaller and harder to find and quite often the hands are of more muscular construction than the feet.

In Chinese reflexology the therapist uses a lot more pressure while doing an exploratory investigation of the area and once they have found a sensitive spot or a spot that gives the patient the most discomfort or pain they will increase the pressure and keep applying more pressure until they find the (life force) "Qi" in the body and ascertain when it is the right intensity. These sessions can be quite painful, but the plus side is they tend to heal more quickly than the slower low pressure style of the Western world.

In Western Reflexology the only things that are used are the hands, usually the finger and thumb tips and sometimes talcum powder is used to stop any slipping (as opposed to a Swedish massage where oil is used to lubricate the hands so they slide easily).

The Chinese style of Reflexology often uses a small roller and a small stick that can help the therapist to feel small grain deposits and locate some of the points.

The differences between reflex points in Chinese and Western Reflexology:

In Chinese reflexology the Heart is below the ball of the foot.
In Western reflexology it is in the center of the left foot.

In Chinese reflexology the Thyroid is located on the ball of the foot.
In Western reflexology it is on the big toe.

In Chinese reflexology the Solar plexus are located in the center.
In Western reflexology they are to one side.

In Chinese reflexology the Stomach is on the inside edge of both feet.
In Western reflexology it is below the ball of the left foot.

In Chinese reflexology the Pancreas is located on the inside edge of both feet.
In Western reflexology it is on the ball of the left foot.

In Chinese reflexology the Liver is located in the outer quadrant of the right foot.
In Western reflexology it is in the large area under the ball of the right foot.

In Chinese reflexology the Bladder is smaller than in Western reflexology.

In Chinese reflexology the Kidney in larger and located in a higher position than in Western reflexology.

In Chinese reflexology the Adrenal is located above the Kidney.
In Western reflexology it is diagonally across and above.

In Chinese reflexology the Sciatic Nerve is located on the edge of the calf.
In Western reflexology it is on the heel of the foot.

In Chinese reflexology the Uterus, Prostrate, Ovary and Testes are located in a large area.
In Western reflexology they are in a much smaller area.

The Spleen is of different shapes.

Western Reflexology is based on the Zone Theory originated by Dr. William Fitzgerald who divided the body into ten zones with the foot also divide into ten corresponding zones. The Chinese Traditional Reflexology is divided into twelve energy meridians or zones, with controlling buttons on the feet that can control the energy or "Qi" of the whole body. Manipulating these buttons and releasing the flow of energy can help the body to relax and recuperate, self-cure or heal itself.

The other main difference is that Western Reflexology is open and easy to learn it practitioners openly teach their patients techniques to enable them to apply it to themselves and indeed it can be learnt in a free course on the internet. In a sharp contrast Chinese Reflexology is a closely guarded secret that is only given to special students and members of the family, it is often handed down from generation to generation and remains within the family. Their Reflexology is surrounded with mystery ceremony and tradition.

Conclusion

Although controversial from a conventional medical perspective, reflexology has helped millions of people around the world – and their numbers keep growing. Since the practice is similar to TCM, which also forms the basis of Japanese and Korean traditional medicine, the governments of those countries have begun subjecting this discipline to scientific scrutiny, again with mixed results.

But for adherents, it doesn't matter what the scientific data has to say on the matter. It works for them, and never mind how. Never mind, as well, what the conventional medical establishment has to say regarding reflexology's claims.

You can, however, take heart in the fact that at least some its claims are supported by the medical evidence. Who knows what else they might say about it in the future?

If you've done the exercises described in this book and assuming they worked for you, then you just might come to the conclusion that there is indeed something to reflexology. If so, then your next step is to find yourself a professional. In America, the government requires all reflexologists to be certified with the

Department of Health, while only North Dakota and Tennessee provide licenses to reflexologists.

To find out if your local reflexologist is indeed certified, head on over to the American Reflexology Certification Board (ARCB) (http://arcb.net/cms/) or to the Reflexology Association of America (RAA) (http://reflexology-usa.org/professionals/). You can also check in with the American Commission for Accreditation for Reflexology Education and Training (ACARET) (http://acaret.org/).

Of those three websites, the RAA has the most comprehensive list and is the one most lay people use to look up reflexologists. It is an independent agency that meets the standards set by the National Commission for Certifying Agencies (NCAA) and the National Organization for Competency Assurance (NOCA).

Keep in mind that this book is a guide to reflexology and cannot possibly cover the practice in its entirety. Its objective is simply to help you understand the basic theory and practice behind the discipline, and to get you started by learning how to self-perform it. But if you'd like to take the next step and learn more, you can also take more in-depth online lessons from the School of Natural Health Sciences (http://www.naturalhealthcourses.com/reflexology.ht

m). For a more comprehensive list of certified schools, visit the Reflexology Schools (http://www.reflexologyschools.org/) website.

Zone therapy was established to provide people with quick, easy-to-do home remedies for common aches and pains. It is in that same spirit that this book is offered.

Thanks for purchasing this book! If you found the information helpful and encouraging, please be so kind as to leave a review for this book on Amazon. Now, go and put everything into practice. You will not be disappointed!

Printed in Great Britain
by Amazon